God's greatest desire is for us to live victorious lives and continually enjoy his blessings bequeathed to us. As God is Spirit & Man also is a Spirit so walk in divine excellence and transform your world through the power of a renewed mind.

Index

1. What is Influenza (Flu)?

2. Flu Symptoms

3. How Flu Spreads

4. How is seasonal incidence of influenza estimated?

5. Does seasonal incidence of influenza change based on the severity of flu season?

6. Complications of Flu

7. How do I know if I have the flu?

8. What kinds of flu tests are there?

9. How well can rapid tests detect the flu?

10. Will my health care provider test me for flu if I have flu-like symptoms?

11. **Most effective Homeopathic medicine for viral influenza.**

12. **Homeopathic selection for a person have both asthma and flu.**

1.   What is Influenza (Flu)?

Going Viral: What to Watch For *Updated April 2, 2020.*

Fever is a common, telltale early symptom of COVID-19, and rare symptoms of the disease typically manifest only in later, severe stages, if at all.

	COLD	FLU	NOROVIRUS	COVID-19*
Incubation period	1-3 days	1-4 days	A few hours	2-14 days
Symptom onset	Gradual	Abrupt	Abrupt	Gradual
Typical illness duration	7-10 days	3-7 days	1-2 days	Undetermined
SYMPTOMS				
Sore throat	Common	Sometimes	Rare	Sometimes
Sneezing	Common	Sometimes	Rare	Rare
Stuffy, runny nose	Common	Sometimes	Rare	Sometimes
Cough, chest discomfort	Sometimes	Common	Rare	Common
Fatigue, weakness	Sometimes	Common	Sometimes	Sometimes
Fever	Rare	Common	Sometimes	Common
Aches	Rare	Common	Sometimes	Sometimes
Chills	Rare	Common	Sometimes	Sometimes
Headache	Rare	Common	Sometimes	Rare
Shortness of breath	Rare	Rare	Rare	Common
Nausea	Rare	Rare	Common	Rare
Vomiting	Rare	Rare	Common	Rare
Diarrhea	Rare	Rare	Common	Rare
Stomach pain	Rare	Rare	Common	Rare

Note: Viruses can be contagious during the incubation period, before symptoms start.

**See below for more detailed information on COVID-19 symptoms.*

SOURCES: Peter Gulick, Michigan State Univ.; CDC; Merck Manual; Univ. of Michigan; Mayo Clinic   GRAPHIC BY ROBERT ROY BRITT

Flu is a contagious respiratory illness caused by influenza viruses that infect the nose, throat, and sometimes the lungs. It can cause mild to severe illness, and at times can lead to death.

2.   Flu Symptoms

Influenza (flu) can cause mild to severe illness, and at times can lead to death. Flu is different from a cold. Flu usually comes on suddenly. People who have flu often feel some or all of these symptoms:

- fever* or feeling feverish/chills
- cough
- sore throat

- runny or stuffy nose

- muscle or body aches

- headaches

- fatigue (tiredness)

- some people may have vomiting and diarrhea, though this is more common in children than adults.

*It's important to note that not everyone with flu will have a fever.

3. How Flu Spreads

Most experts believe that flu viruses spread mainly by tiny droplets made when people with flu cough, sneeze or talk. These droplets can land in the mouths or noses of people who are nearby. Less often, a person might get flu by touching a surface or object that has flu virus on it and then touching their own mouth, nose or possibly their eyes.

How Many People Get Sick with Flu Every Year?

A 2018 CDC study published in Clinical Infectious Diseasesexternal icon looked at the percentage of the U.S. population who were sickened by flu using two different methods and compared the findings. Both methods had similar findings, which suggested that on average, about 8% of the U.S. population gets sick from flu each season, with a range of between 3% and 11%, depending on the season.

Why is the 3% to 11% estimate different from the previously cited 5% to 20% range?

The commonly cited 5% to 20% estimate was based on a study that examined both symptomatic and asymptomatic influenza illness, which means it also looked at people who may have had the flu but never knew it because they didn't have any symptoms. The 3% to 11% range is an estimate of the proportion of people who have symptomatic flu illness.

Who is most likely to be infected with influenza?

The same CID studyexternal icon found that children are most likely to get sick from flu and that people 65 and older are least likely to get sick from influenza. Median incidence values (or attack rate) by age group were 9.3% for children 0-17 years, 8.8% for adults 18-64 years, and 3.9% for adults 65 years and older. This means that children younger than 18 are more than twice as likely to develop a symptomatic flu infection than adults 65 and older.

4. **How is seasonal incidence of influenza estimated?**

Influenza virus infection is so common that the number of people infected each season can only be estimated. These statistical estimations are based on <u>CDC-measured flu hospitalization rates</u> that are adjusted to produce an estimate of the total number of influenza infections in the United States for a given flu season.

The estimates for the number of infections are then divided by the census population to estimate the seasonal incidence (or attack rate) of influenza.

5. Does seasonal incidence of influenza change based on the severity of flu season?

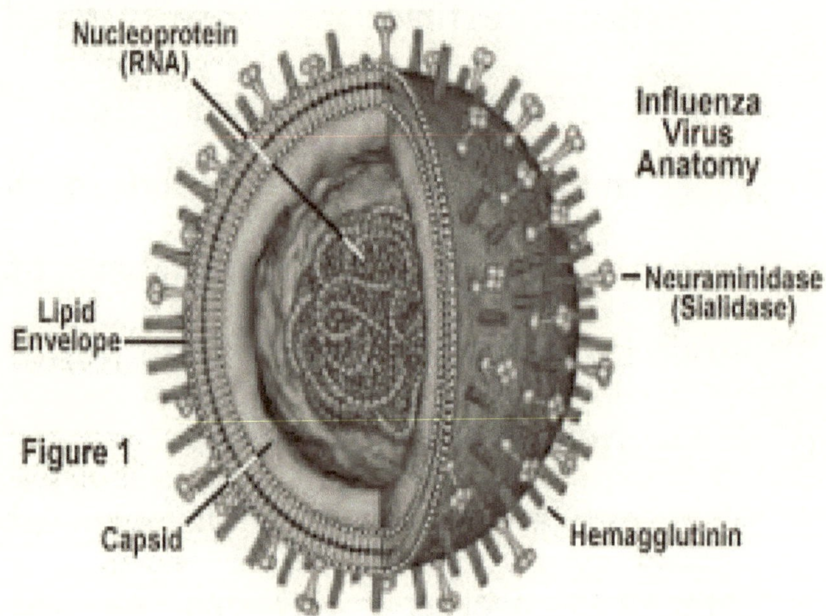

Yes. The proportion of people who get sick from flu varies. A paper published in CID external icon found that between 3% and 11% of the U.S. population gets infected and develops flu symptoms each year. The 3% estimate is from the 2011-2012 season, which was an H1N1-predominant season classified as being of low severity. The estimated incidence of flu illness during two seasons was around 11%; 2012-2013 was an H3N2-predominant season classified as being of moderate severity, while 2014-2015 was an H3N2 predominant season classified as being of high severity.

Table 1. Estimates of the Incidence of Symptomatic Influenza by Season and Age-Group, United States, 2010-2016

Season	Predominant Virus(es)	Season Severity	Season Incidence, %, by Age Group					
			0-	5-	18	50	≥6	All

			4 yrs	17 yrs	- 49 yrs	- 64 yrs	5 yrs	Ages
2010 -11	A/H3N2, A/H1N1pdm 09	Modera te	14. 1	8.4	5.3	8.1	4.3	6.8
2011 -12	A/H3N2	Low	4.8	3.6	2.5	3.1	2.3	3.0
2012 -13	A/H3N2	Modera te	18. 6	12. 7	8.9	14. 3	9.9	11.3
2013 -14	A/H1N1pdm 09	Modera te	12. 4	7.2	9.2	13. 0	3.4	9.0
2014 -15	A/H3N2	High	15 0	12. 7	7.8	12. 9	12. 4	10.8
2015 -16	A/H1N1pdm 09	Modera te	11.1	7.4	7.1	11. 0	3.5	7.6
Media n			13. 2	7.9	7.4	12. 0	3.9	8.3

Period of Contagiousness

You may be able to spread flu to someone else before you know you are sick, as well as while you are sick.

- People with flu are most contagious in the first 3-4 days after their illness begins.
- Some otherwise healthy adults may be able to infect others beginning 1 day **before** symptoms develop and up to 5 to 7 days **after** becoming sick.
- Some people, especially young children and people with weakened immune systems, might be able to

infect others for an even longer time.

Onset of Symptoms

The time from when a person is exposed and infected with flu to when symptoms begin is about 2 days, but can range from about 1 to 4 days.

6.Complications of Flu

Complications of flu can include bacterial pneumonia, ear infections, sinus infections and worsening of chronic medical conditions, such as congestive heart failure, asthma, or diabetes.

People at High Risk from Flu.

Anyone can get flu (even healthy people), and serious problems related to flu can happen at any age, but some people are at high risk of developing serious flu-related complications if they get sick. This includes people 65 years and older, people of any age with certain chronic medical conditions (such as asthma, diabetes, or heart disease), pregnant women, and children younger than 5 years.

7.How do I know if I have the flu?

Your respiratory illness might be the flu if you have fever, cough, sore throat, runny or stuffy nose, body aches, headache, chills and fatigue. Some people may have vomiting and diarrhea. People may be infected with the flu and have respiratory symptoms without a fever. Flu viruses usually cause the most illness during the colder months of the year. However, influenza can also occur outside of the typical flu season. In addition, other viruses can also cause respiratory illness similar to the flu. So, it is impossible to tell for sure if you have the flu based on symptoms alone. If your doctor needs to know for sure whether you have the flu, there are laboratory tests that can be done.

8. What kinds of flu tests are there?

A number of flu tests are available to detect influenza viruses in respiratory specimens. The most common are called "rapid influenza diagnostic tests (RIDTs)." RIDTs work by detecting the parts of the virus (antigens) that stimulate an immune response. These tests can provide results within approximately 10-15 minutes, but are not as accurate as other flu tests. Therefore, you could still have the flu, even though your rapid test result is negative. Other flu tests are called "rapid molecular assays" that detect genetic material of the virus. Rapid molecular assays produce results in 15-20 minutes and are more accurate than RIDTs. In addition, there are several more-accurate and sensitive flu tests available that must be performed in specialized laboratories, such as those found in hospitals or state public health laboratories. All of these tests require that a health care provider swipe the inside of your nose or the back of your throat with a swab and then send the swab for testing. Results may take one hour or several hours.

9. How well can rapid tests detect the flu?

During an influenza outbreak, a positive rapid flu test is likely to indicate influenza infection. However, rapid tests vary in their ability to detect flu viruses, depending on the type of rapid test used, and on the type of flu viruses circulating. Also, rapid tests appear to be better at detecting flu in children than adults. This variation in ability to detect viruses can result in some people who are infected with the flu having a negative rapid test result. (This situation is called a false negative test result.) Despite a negative rapid test result, your health care provider may diagnose you with flu based on your symptoms and their clinical judgment.

10. Will my health care provider test me for flu if I have flu-like symptoms?

Not necessarily. Most people with flu symptoms are not tested because the test results usually do not change how you are treated.

Your health care provider may diagnose you with flu based on your symptoms and their clinical judgment or they may choose to use an influenza diagnostic test. During an outbreak of respiratory illness, testing for flu can help determine if flu viruses are the cause of the outbreak. Flu testing can also be helpful for some people with suspected flu who are pregnant or have a weakened immune system, and for whom a diagnosis of flu can help their doctor make decisions about their care.

11. Most effective Homeopathic Selection.

Combination – I (Prevention from Viral flu)

1. Influenzium -30
2. Aconite – 30

3. Eupatorium perfoliatum -30

4. Arsenic album – 30

> **Mix each of the above 4 medicine in equal amount into a glass bottle and take 2 drops in the morning after every 2 days.**

Take globules bottle as given in image.

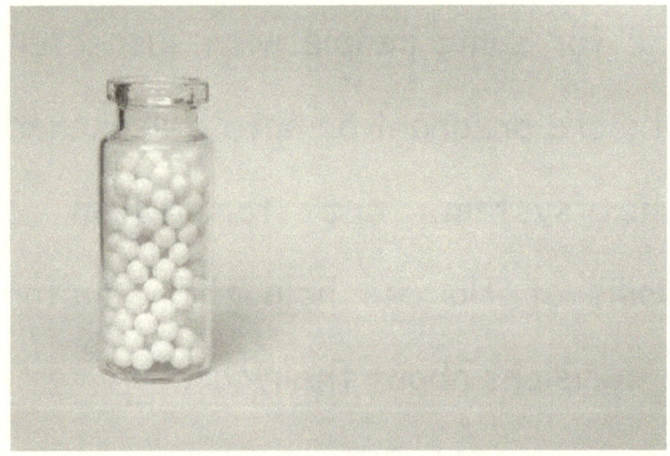

Mix 4 - 5 drops of each of the above 1, 2, 3, and 4 medicine into 20 ml of globules bottle and take 4 – 6 globules 2 or 3 times a day during flu (influenza) season. It develop immunity against flu and protect our body in getting more infective.

Note:- Orange Juice and Coconut Water are most effective immune booster against any viral infection.

Dose:- Take your body weight multiply by 9 gram above juice daily.

- If Body weight is 70 Kg, Dose will be 630 Gram.
- If Body weight is 60 Kg, Dose will be 540 Gram.

Combination – II (Flue treatment)

Type – A (Compulsory)

1. Ocimim Sanctum – Q

2. Tinospora Cordifolia – Q

3. China Officinalis – Q

4. Echinacea – Q

Mix 20 ml of each into a glass bottle and take 15 to 20 drops 3 times a day with half cup of water.

Type – B   (Optional Medicine in case of fever)

1. Chirata – Q
2. Baptisia – Q

> Mix 20 ml of each into a gloass bottle and take 15 drops 3 times a day with half cup of water after 50 minute of Type – A combination in case of fever.

Type – C (Compulsory)

1. Influenzium -30
2. Aconite – 30
3. Eupatorium perfoliatum -30

4. Arsenic album – 30

5. Allum Cepa -30

Mix each of the above 5 medicine in equal amount into a glass bottle and take 3 drops 3 times a day.

Combination : III (Lungs Congestion)

Type-A (Compulsory)

1. Natrum Mur – 30

2. Eupatorium perfoliatum – 30

3. Merc sol - 30

4. Aconitum – 30

Mix all the above 4 medicine in equal amount into a glass bottle and take 3 drops 3 times a day.

Type – B (Compulsory)

1. Hepar Suph – 200

2. Aconite – 200

3. Spongia tosta – 200

Mix all the above 3 medicine in equal amount into a glass bottle and take 3 drops 3 times a day after 15 minutes of Type – A medicine.

Type – C (Compulsory)

1. Ipecacuanha – 30

2. Antimonium Tartaricum -30

>   **Mix all the above 2 medicine in equal amount into a glass bottle and take 3 drops 3 times a day after 15 minutes of Type – B medicine.**

Type – D (Compulsory or optional as per symptoms)

Take 8 ml of Wheezal Mixture for adult and 2.5 to 4 ml of Wheezal Mixture for children after 15 minutes of Type -c medicine.

Note;- In case of asthmatic symptoms or a patient have both asthma and flu then he should take flu medicine with asthma treatment as mentioned below.

- ## **Homeopathic combination for asthma.**

Combination: - I

Type-A

1. **Blatta Orientalis Q (60 %)**
2. **Pothos Q (20 %)**
3. **Grindelia Q (20 %)**

   Mix all of the above liquid into a bottle and takes 20 drops 3 times a day with half cup of water.

Type-B

1. **Sulphur 30 or Calcarea Carbonicum 30   (Choose any one of the above as per your body structure or symptoms). --   2 Drops morning daily taking one day gap after every 7 days**
2. **Arelia rasimosa 30 (2 Drops 3 times a day)**

3. Bio Combination 2 (4 Pills 3 times a day)

(Take Both Type A and Type B medicine

as suggested above)

Combination – II (Most effective)

Type-A

1. Blatta Orientalis Q

2. Ipecacuanha Inflata Q

3. Grindeia Robusta Q

4. Justicia Adhatoda Q

5. Senega Q

6. Lobelia Inflata Q

7. Bio Combination 2 (4 Pills 3 times a day)

Mix No. 1, 2 and 3 in equal amount into a bottle and take 20 drops 3 times a day with half cup of water.

Mix No. 4, 5 and 6 in equal amount into a bottle and take 20 drops 3 times a day with half cup of water.

Note:- You can replace above Combination-II by Asthamin Homeopathic syrup and take 1 spoon 3 times a day.

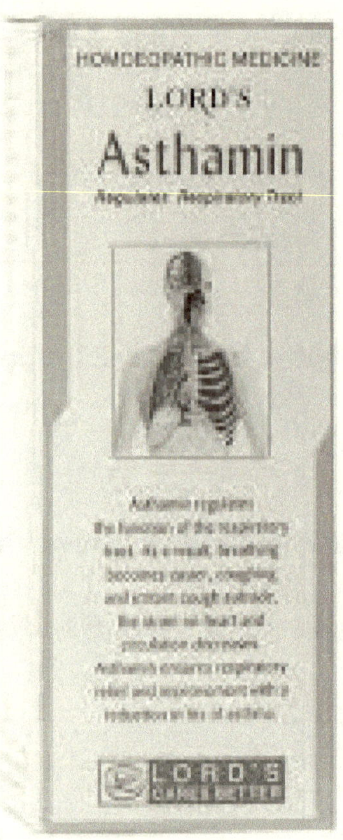

Note:-   Choose Only one Combination – I   or Combination – II of the above.

Thanking You.